KILL VIRUSES NOW

Jack D. Warner

Copyright © 2020 Jack D. Warner

All Rights Reserved

No part of this publication may be reproduced, stored, or transmitted in any form or by any means, electronic, mechanical, photocopying, recording, scanning, or otherwise without written permission from the publisher. It is illegal to copy this book, post it to a website, or distribute it by any other means without permission.

Medical Disclaimer

The information in any of our handouts, e-books, written material, whether provided in hardcopy or digitally (together 'Material') is for general information purposes and nothing contained in it is, or is intended to be construed as advice. It does not take into account your individual health, medical, physical or emotional situation or needs. It is not a substitute for medical attention, treatment, examination, advice, treatment of existing conditions or diagnosis and is not intended to provide a clinical diagnosis nor take the place of proper medical advice from a fully qualified medical practitioner. You should, before you act or use any of this information, consider the appropriateness of this information having regard to your own personal situation and needs. You are responsible for consulting a suitable medical professional before using any of the information or materials contained in our Material or accessed through our website, before trying any treatment or taking any course of action that may directly or indirectly affect your health or well-being.

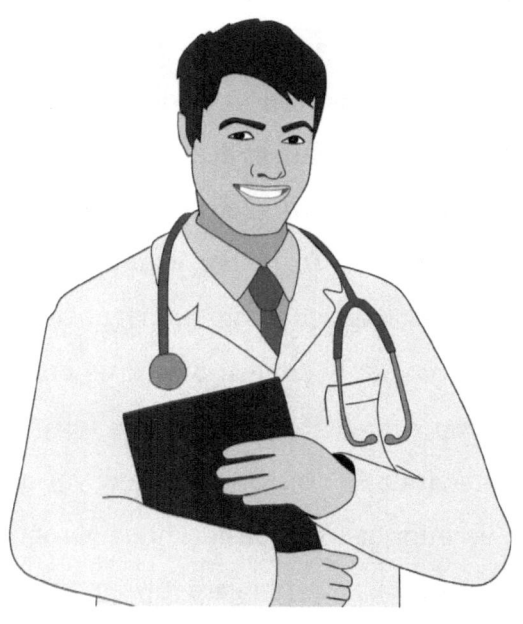

Dedication

This book is dedicated to the Health and Wellness of humanity!

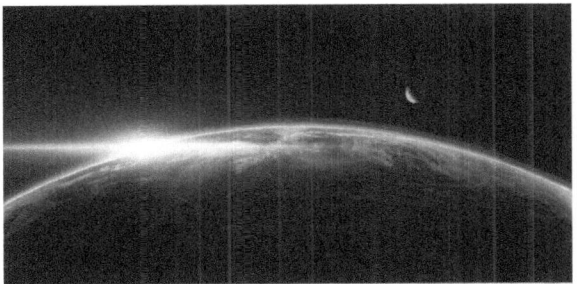

Epigraph

"Life is a succession of lessons which must be lived to be understood."

— Ralph Waldo Emerson

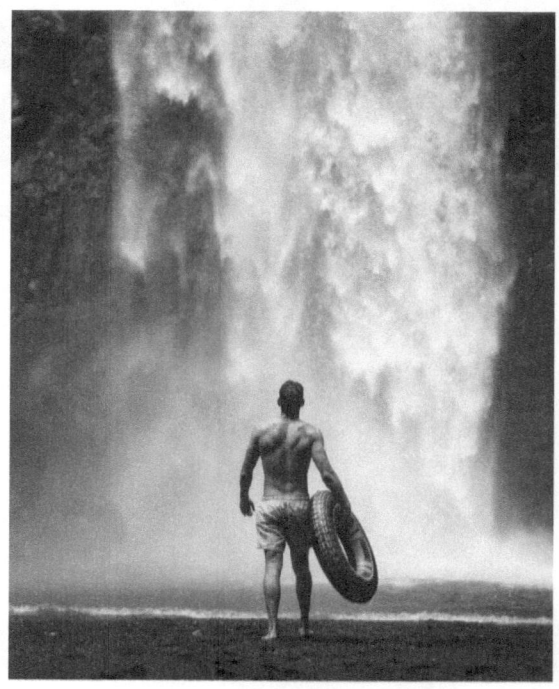

Table of Contents

Preface 1

Introduction 5

  Medical Ozone 11

    What Is Ozone? 12

    Ozone As The Virus Killer 12

    The History Of Ozone Therapy 13

    How Does Ozone Therapy Work? 14

    What Are The Other Benefits Of Ozone Therapy? 14

    How Is Ozone Administered To The Body? ... 15

    Treatment Preferences 18

    Worldwide Usage Of Ozone Therapy 18

  Colloidal Ionic Hydrosol Silver 23

    What Is Colloidal Silver And Who Has Used It? 24

- What Is The Safest Form Of Colloidal Silver? 24
- Dosing Reference By The Usepa 25
- Colloidal Silver Dosage 26
- My Silver Hydrosol Healing Protocol 26
- What Is The Effect Of Colloidal Silver On The Human Body? 27
- How Long Does It Take For Colloidal Silver To Kill A Virus? 28

Vitamin C - Oral 34
- What Is Vitamin C? 35
- How Does Vitamin C Function? 37
- How Many Types Of Vitamin C Are There? .. 37
- Which Form Of Vitamin C Is Best? 38
- Extra Benefits Of Taking Oral Vitamin C 39

Vitamin C - Intravenous 41
- Vitamin C Against Viral Infection 42
- Worldwide Clinical Trials 43

- Antiviral Herbs List 50
  - Most Common Antiviral Herbs: 51
- Antiviral Supplements 60
  - The Most Studied Supplements For Their Effectiveness In Preventing And Treating Viral Infections. 61
- Antiviral Food 66
- Immune Boosting Juices 73
- Nitric Oxide(No) 78
  - What Is Nitric Oxide? 79
  - How Does Nitric Oxide Help The Body? 79
  - How Can We Supply The Body With Nitric Oxide? 80
- Coming Soon - Volume 2 88
- Coming Soon - Volume 3 90

Kill Viruses Now

PREFACE

Jack D. Warner

This Health & Wellness Series would not have been written without the prodding of my friends, and physicians. I have been asked by many about the details of my daily protocols. They thought I must have stumbled upon the fountain of youth where vibrant health, longevity, and youthfulness abounded. It is true that I look, act, and feel much younger than my biological age with energy that is usually reserved for the very young. Do I really have the secrets to vibrant eternal youth? I might have. That is the topic of volume 2 in this series, namely "Perfect De-Aging" as well as volume 3 titled "Incredible Shakes of the Gods". But for now, I will proceed by sharing with you my disease-free protocols that I believe have saved me over decades from catastrophic illnesses including viral infections.

I had been an individual who was born with a weak immune system. I was the victim of constant bouts of all kinds of inflammations and infections including severe colds and influenza. Thanks to all the practical knowledge that I have learned from all the scientific research I feel that I have now achieved near total immunity from opportunistic immune attackers including viruses. Thus, I have chosen to begin my volume 1 of Health and Wellness Series with "Kill Viruses Now".

My decision has risen from the fact that any viral infections should not be taken lightly. As I have successfully done during the last few decades, I believe that clearing the body from all virus-causing diseases should be done at the onset of viral attacks. They must be stripped from their ability to mutate, to become drug-resistant, or even transform themselves into newer and more deadly forms. Could this existential threat to humans be stopped in its tracks? The emphatic answer that seems to come from other research scientists is a resounding YES!

This is what my book is poised to reveal to the world. This is the real and practical account of many of my protocols that I have been applying for a long time.

Yes, I no longer live in fear of any attacking viruses or pathogens. The different protocols that I have been following seem to have produced an immune system that is the envy of people of all ages including my much revered and beloved physicians.

PS. This book is not attempting to report on all the research into overcoming viral diseases, General references have only been furnished here for your further research purposes. I am merely trying to prove that the self-made protocols that I have been following for very long time seem to have at last been vindicated according to all the scientific studies including the ones that are mentioned in the reference sections.

Kill Viruses Now

INTRODUCTION

A few years ago, I happened to catch a seemingly very bad cold. At that time, I was not applying my protocols prophylactically. So, I thought it would be a good idea to go to the emergency room for a checkup before I consider applying any of my healing protocols on myself. Upon checking myself into the emergency room, one of the doctors on call decided to have me admitted to the hospital for further testing. I was concerned about the doctor's decision, but I went along and decided to follow the doctor's advice.

The shocker came when a nurse donning a surgical mask and carrying a clipboard entered my hospital room. She wanted to know what kind of authorization I would give the hospital in case of a lung collapse and eventual death. To my surprise I immediately came to the realization that the doctor had concluded that I had pneumonia. Obviously, the supervising doctor at the time had a very dim chance of my surviving it.

Luckily, I remembered that I had in my backpack a glass dropper bottle full of the substance that is mentioned in this book under the name of PROTOCOL 2. Upon knowing of the dire situation that I was in, I immediately started taking two dropperful sublingual dose of that substance every two hours during the night while at the same time I was being connected to an overnight IV. The next morning the doctor came in and ordered more x-rays of my lungs. To her surprise she informed me that the pneumonia had mysteriously vanished. At that moment I was relieved and delighted after the subsequent additional x-rays which confirmed my sudden recovery that ended up with my subsequent release from the hospital.

I remember not telling the doctor about my emergency treatment that I performed on myself because I did not want that doctor to start investigating my sudden recovery. But later, my primary physician was supportive after I informed him of the hospitalization incident and my seemingly miraculous recovery.

After my discharge from the hospital that morning, I decided to start taking prophylactic measures to ensure my freedom from diseases before they strike. I now believe for sure that at least one of my protocols has saved me from dying a terrible pneumonic death at the hospital.

During the subsequent years I fervently started taking the invaluable scientific knowledge of my PRORTOCOLS very seriously after my last emergency encounter. Ever since that scary incident at the hospital I never had any reason to go back. I feel that I am now in control of any health problems that may suddenly arise. I realize that I do have all the means that I need to protect myself effectively and safely in my own home and/or at a Holistic Clinic. Of course, I still go to my primary and specialist doctors for periodical diagnostics lab tests to make sure that I am successful in maintaining super healthy existence.

It is worth mentioning that during my routine health checkup visits to my doctors, I happened to find out that they had gotten increasingly curious and wanted to know more details about my newly found immunity. I suddenly seemed to them to have gotten stronger, younger looking and healthier than before. Some of them started calling me names. I seemed to have become the "boy wonder" to most of them. Even my primary doctor told me that he had been proudly using the "boy wonder" nickname that he gave me in order to prove his point during his teaching sessions to newly hired doctors. He told me that he was talking about me as the perfect patient who has successfully gotten involved in designing natural safe treatments for himself.

This is big news to have a teaching doctor acknowledging my successful application of natural medicine instead or/and in conjunction with any needed prescription drugs. This physician and other doctors were the ones who have encouraged me to share my experiences in healing myself by writing a book about it. They uncharacteristically believed that there is always a place for alternative medicine. This is how my book has gotten its inspiration and its inception.

PS. Please be aware that I am not against taking lifesaving drugs if and when needed.

Kill Viruses Now

PROTOCOL 1

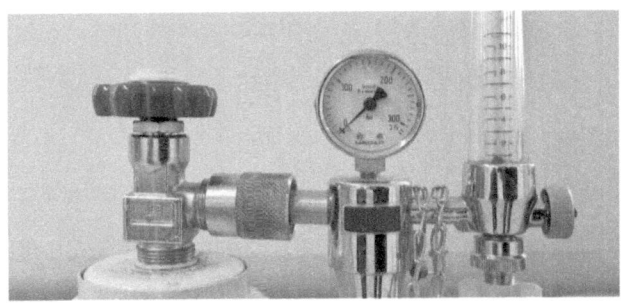

MEDICAL OZONE.

What is Ozone?

Ozone, or O3, is a gas consisting of three atoms of oxygen. O3 is different from the oxygen that is needed to breathe, which is known as O2 and consists of two atoms. Because Ozone (O3) has three oxygen atoms, it can be useful as an agent of reaction. Essentially, in order to achieve the more stable form, an Ozone molecule would volunteer to give away an atom of oxygen—a process called oxidation. The free oxygen atom has the ability to combine and alter other substances, which is the basis for Ozone's reactivity,

Ozone as the virus killer.

The US National Library of Medicine supplies the ongoing Clinical Trials results of using Ozone Therapy in the fight against the latest viruses. They mention that Ozone Therapy has become a promising treatment for both prevention and treatment of viral infections. The oxidative stress created by Ozone in the body has very positive results such as:

1. Stimulating the peripheral phagocytic cells.

2. Activation of the antioxidant system.

3. Restoring the immune system.

The History of Ozone Therapy

Ozone therapy is not new. It has been in use since the 1800's. The famous inventor Nikola Tesla patented his first ozone generator in 1896. It was registered in the United States under the name of Tesla Ozone Company.

In the 1980s German physicians had successfully been treating HIV and cancer patients with ozone. A lot of ongoing clinical trials around the world have been investigating the effectiveness of Ozone therapy.

How Does Ozone Therapy work?

Ozone is effective on multiple levels and could definitely have a detrimental effect on virus-infected cells. It actually starts deactivating and killing viruses within 6 minutes. The "killing" process takes place as soon as the Ozone is introduced to the body.

1. It damages and disrupts the integrity of the cell envelope.

2. It oxidizes the phospholipids and lipoproteins in the cells.

3. It causes the inactivation and paralysis of the virus in the infected cells.

4. It safely removes the damaged infected cells after being inactivated by the presence of Ozone.

What are the other benefits of Ozone Therapy?

Ozone is known to have the following positive effects on the body:

1. Strengthens the immune system by stimulating white blood cells.

2. Prevents infections.

3. Counteracts cell mutations thus preventing any type of deadly diseases.

How is ozone administered to the body?

There are many methods of administering Ozone. The first method is given through specialized clinics that operate in many countries around the world including the United States of America. For example, one can have a medical professional in his/her city administer the Ozone according to the health care professional's prescription. It could be administered intravenously at the clinic or at home for treatment of any infection that is caused by any viruses. Also, Ozone treatments could be administered through rectal insufflation, through the ears, and through the mouth by drinking the ozonated water. These treatments could be given daily or weekly as needed until the desired results are achieved. Ozone treatments are usually performed at alternative medical clinics which might offer different traditional and non-traditional therapies.

1. Homeopathic traditional medicine

2. Chiropractic, and acupuncture

3. Complementary medicine clinics which use combined treatments with conventional medicine.

4. Ozone clinics that are operated by doctors.

The following is a summary of methods that those clinics use to administer the Ozone gas into the body:

1. Rectum

2. Vagina

3. Intramuscular

4. Subcutaneous

5. Intravenous

6. Autohemotherapy

7. Mouth

8. Ear

Ozone therapy at home is done by administering some of the above-mentioned treatments in complete privacy but under the supervision of a healthcare professional.

Different varieties of Ozone generators are also readily available for sale anywhere on this planet. The pricing depends on the types of the Ozone generators that range in price from a few dollars to thousands of dollars. For prophylactic or ongoing Ozone treatments, I have had great results by using a $40 ozonator machine that I use at home in complete privacy.

PS. Never inhale Ozone gas. Always operate the ozone therapy equipment in well-ventilated areas while making the ozonated water. I usually use a clean washcloth to cover the glass of water while the water is being ozonated. I usually drink that water after a lapse of 30 minutes once or twice a day on an empty stomach as needed. Also there are Ozone accessories that are sold on websites where Ozone equipment are sold.

Treatment Preferences

The first choice is to get Ozone therapy in a clinic. The clinic can provide more therapy choices, and administer it in a safe, professional environment. It is recommended that one should consult a physician before attempting any Ozone therapy at home!

Worldwide usage of Ozone Therapy

Clinicaltrials.gov mentions that China and Italy were among the few Asian and European countries to conduct several studies that analyzed the mechanisms by which Ozone Therapy could combat viral infections. These are the results of the benefits noted in the various studies:

1. Improvement of the release of oxygen in the peripheral tissues.

2. Anti-inflammatory action

3. Virucidal activity

The studies also mention that during the use of Ozone Therapy, probiotic supplementation should be given to the patients to correct any issues that are connected to the intestinal microbiome.

GENERAL REFERENCES:

Hernández A, Papadakos PJ, Torres A, González DA, Vives M, Ferrando C, Baeza J. Two known therapies could be useful as adjuvant therapy in critical patients infected by COVID-19. Rev Esp Anestesiol Reanim. 2020 May;67(5):245-252. doi: 10.1016/j.redar.2020.03.004. Epub 2020 Apr 14. English, Spanish.

Conti P, Gallenga CE, Tetè G, Caraffa A, Ronconi G, Younes A, Toniato E, Ross R, Kritas SK. How to reduce the likelihood of coronavirus-19 (CoV-19 or SARS-CoV-2) infection and lung inflammation mediated by IL-1. J Biol Regul Homeost Agents. 2020 Mar 31;34(2). doi: 10.23812/Editorial-Conti-2.

Cascella M, Rajnik M, Cuomo A, Dulebohn SC, Di Napoli R. Features, Evaluation and Treatment Coronavirus (COVID-19). 2020 May 18. StatPearls [Internet]. Treasure Island (FL): StatPearls Publishing; 2020 Jan-.
http://www.ncbi.nlm.nih.gov/books/NBK554776/

Xu K, Cai H, Shen Y, Ni Q, Chen Y, Hu S, Li J, Wang H, Yu L, Huang H, Qiu Y, Wei G, Fang Q, Zhou J, Sheng J, Liang T, Li L. [Management of corona virus disease-19 (COVID-19): the Zhejiang experience]. Zhejiang Da Xue Xue Bao Yi Xue Ban. 2020 Feb 21;49(1):0. Chinese.

https://www.ncbi.nlm.nih.gov/pmc/articles/PMC3312702/

https://www.epa.gov/indoor-air-quality-iaq/ozone-generators-aresold-aircleaners# intro

http://www.ozonesolutions.com/info/ozone-faq

http://drsozone.com/medical-info/3-page-intro/

http://www.rice.edu/~jenky/sports/antiox.html

http://www.wimbledonclinic.co.uk/documents/Ozonetherapyasantioxidant.pdf

https://www.cancer.gov/publications/dictionaries/cancerterms?cdrid=45256

https://www.naturopathicgroup.com/iv-nutrient-therapy/iv-ozone.html

http://drsozone.com/medical-info/safety-side-effects/

https://www.ncbi.nlm.nih.gov/pmc/articles/PMC3298518/

http://drsozone.com/medical-info/contraindications/
R

Kill Viruses Now

PROTOCOL 2

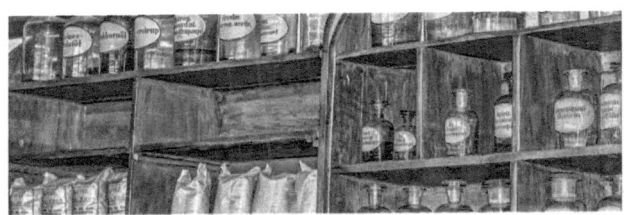

COLLOIDAL IONIC HYDROSOL SILVER

What is colloidal silver and who has used it?

Silver is a natural element that is found in everyday food such as whole grains, mushrooms, milk, and even water. It has been used medicinally throughout the ages. History books mention that the ancient Greek physician Hippocrates wrote about silver's healing and anti-disease properties. Colloidal silver was a preferred choice of physicians in the 1930s. NASA has used colloidal silver to purify drinking water on the International Space Station.

What is the safest form of colloidal silver?

There are many forms of colloidal silver on the market. Ingesting poorly produced silver with contaminations could result in what is called Argyria - a condition of blue discoloration of the skin. For myself, I make sure to choose products that are free of proteins, salts, or any other compounds. The safest form of silver is the one that has 10 PPM with 99.999% pure homeopathic silver that is packaged in amber colored glass bottles which are crucial to ensure the stability and quality of hydrosol silver.

Dosing Reference by the USEPA

A dosing reference created by the United States Environmental Protection Agency suggests that the daily silver exposure, topical, oral, or environmental should not exceed 5 micrograms per every kilogram of weight.

The dosage should be administered under the tongue. The product label usually recommends placing drops of colloidal silver under the tongue for 30 or 60 seconds on a clean mouth. It further recommends taking the silver drops half an hour before eating or drinking anything other than pure water and about one or two hours after eating or drinking coffee, tea, soda. etc. There is usually some information on the product label that explains how to administer the colloidal silver for the different conditions and the right dosage for each.

Colloidal Silver Dosage

The dosage should be held under the tongue for about 60 seconds before swallowing.

1. Adults are advised to take one teaspoon dosage or two dropperful of liquid silver.

2. Children are to be given half a teaspoon dosage or one dropperful of silver solution.

Since colloidal silver is a potent antiviral agent, probiotic supplementation after usage is usually recommended to maintain a proper balance of microbiome in the intestines.

My Silver Hydrosol Healing Protocol

a. Once daily for maintenance.

b. Three times daily for immune building.

c. Five times daily for long-term immune support.

d. Seven times daily for short-term immune support.

What is the effect of colloidal silver on the human body?

Health authority Dr Robert O. Becker, MD reported in his book, "The Body Electric" that colloidal silver has miraculous effect on the body.

1. Accelerates the healing process by over 50%.

2. Kills disease-causing viruses within minutes.

3. Facilitates major growth stimulation of injured tissues.

4. Heals human fibroblast cells of organs and tissues in patients over the age of 50 as rapidly as seen naturally in much younger people.

5. Kills viruses in 1 to 6 minutes upon contact.

6. The disease-causing viruses has no time to mutate into a resistant strain.

How long does it take for colloidal silver to kill a virus?

The duration takes only six minutes. The following is the fascinating process that happens to struggling virus infected cells in the human body. Here is a simplified description of this process:

1. A virus decides to invade a living cell of body tissue.

2. It starts to take over the nucleus of the cell.

3. The cell gets transformed into a more primitive enzymatic structure thus altering its reproductive mechanism.

4. The virus takes advantage of this transformation and starts replicating itself through the infected cells.

5. If left unchecked, the virus ends up replicating millions of infected cells which end up in one's bloodstream.

6. Colloidal silver is introduced sublingually.

7. Within 6 minutes of the ingestion of colloidal silver, the infected cell itself becomes a hostile host to the virus.

8. The virus is immediately and permanently disabled, paralyzed, and eventually dies.

9. Finally, the body disposes of the remnants of infected cells.

10. This batch of cells would find their way out of the body through the daily natural disposal of the millions of cells that have ended their usefulness.

11. If the colloidal silver kills the viruses faster than the body can eliminate them, a flu-like symptom might appear.

12. This condition is called the Healing Crisis and should dissipate fast by drinking plenty of

water in order to flush the dead viruses out of the body.

There are a lot of other advantages of taking colloidal silver for diseases like AIDS and cancer. I will leave it up to the reader to discover them by conducting a search on the internet regarding other usages of colloidal silver.

The FDA has stated that because colloidal silver is accepted as a pre-1938 medication, it may continue to be marketed. On September 13, 1991, a document discussed the above fact was published by the consumer safety officer Harold Davis, U.S. Food and Drug Administration titled "Colloidal Preparations of Silver in Pharmacy."

The British Medical Journal mentioned that Pure Silver is entirely non-irritant in tests at very high concentrations and that it has been shown repeatedly that the rapidly exerted disinfectant action is of considerable therapeutic value.

Kill Viruses Now

GENERAL REFERENCES:

The End of Miracle Drugs? Newsweek Magazine, March 28, 1994 Antibiotics

The Ebola Outbreak of 1995 Newsweek Magazine, May 22,1995."

Ions, Atoms and Charged Particles By Francis S. Key and George Maass, PhD

Mechanisms of Silver Nanoparticle Release, Transformation and Toxicity: A Critical Review of Current Knowledge and Recommendations for Future Studies and Applications

Silver Nanoparticles: No Threat to the Environment by George J. Maass, Ph.D.

Colloidal Silver - The Rediscovery of a Super Antibiotic?.

World Without Cancer by G. Edward Griffin - History of allopathic medicine in America.

Chemistry's Miraculous Colloids by Kenneth Andrews. The Readers Digest, March 1936. Quoting, Dr. Frederick Macy, one of the country's outstanding bacteriologists.

John Hopkins Hospital, More News on Silver. Dr. Leonard Herschberg.

Colloidal Silver: Where Does it go when you drink it? How long does it stay there? by Roger Altman Eng. Sc. D.

Searle, A.B. The use of Colloids in Health and Disease. The British Medical Journal. Nov, 1913, p. 83 Dr. Henry Crookes.

Antibacterial efficacy of colloidal silver alone and in combination with other antibiotics on isolates from wound Infections Iroha, I. R1, Esimone, C. O.2, Orji J. O.1 and Imomoh, O. O.

Jack D. Warner

PROTOCOL 3

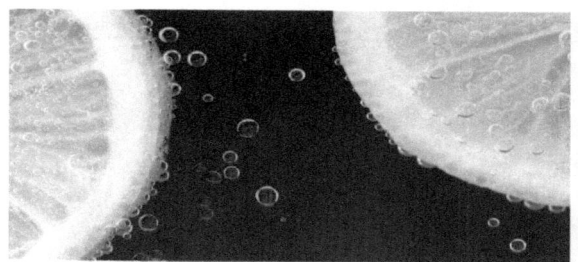

VITAMIN C - ORAL

What is vitamin C?

Vitamin C, which is known as L-ascorbic acid, is a water-soluble vitamin. Unlike most mammals and other animals, humans do not have the ability to synthesize vitamin C and must obtain it from the diet or supplements. Since its discovery in 1928, vitamin C has been known to have a positive effect on the various functions inside the human body:

1. It helps in the development and maintenance of connective tissues.

2. It plays an important role in bone formation.

3. It accelerates wound healing.

4. It helps in the maintenance of healthy gums.

   Vitamin C also plays an important role in a number of important metabolic functions:

1. It helps in the activation of the B vitamin and folic acid.

2. It plays an important role in the conversion of cholesterol to bile acids.

3. It helps in the conversion of the amino acid, tryptophan, to the neurotransmitter, serotonin.

4. It is an antioxidant that protects the body from free radical damage.

5. It is used as a therapeutic agent in many diseases and disorders.

6. It also protects the immune system.

7. It reduces the severity of allergic reactions.

8. It helps to fight off viral infections.

How does Vitamin C function?

Vitamin C (L-ascorbic acid) is a potent reducing agent, meaning that it readily donates electrons to recipient molecules. Related to this oxidation-reduction (redox) potential, two major functions of vitamin C are as an antioxidant and as an enzyme cofactor.

Vitamin C exerts its antiviral properties by:

1. Supporting lymphocyte activity
2. Increasing interferon-α production
3. Modulating cytokines
4. Reducing inflammation
5. Improving endothelial dysfunction
6. Restoring mitochondrial function

How many types of vitamin C are there?

1. Rapid release capsules, tablets, and powder.

2. Time-release capsules and tablets promote delayed and continual absorption throughout the day. These capsules are surrounded by a semi-permeable coating, blended with fats and waxes. When swallowed, moisture from saliva causes the coating to slowly rupture and the vitamin C is continually delivered into the body's fluids over an extended period of time.

3. Liposomal C gel capsules or liquid is sodium ascorbate made of essential phospholipids that transport the vitamin into the bloodstream and the cells microscopically. In other words, liposomal Vitamin C offers a better way to absorb Vitamin C.

Which form of vitamin C is best?

1. It is usually advised to take the rapid release form of vitamin C for immediate results.

2. The time release form of vitamin C has been known for its protective effect in the large intestines against cancer.

Extra benefits of taking oral vitamin C

1. It plays an essential factor on the Antiviral Immune Responses through the production of Interferon-α/β

2. Boosts immunity.

3. Lowers the risk of heart disease.

4. Manages high blood pressure.

5. Normalizes blood uric acid levels.

6. Prevents gout attacks.

7. Provides protection against viral infections

8. Reduces both the physical and psychological effects of stress on people.

Jack D. Warner

Kill Viruses Now

PROTOCOL 4

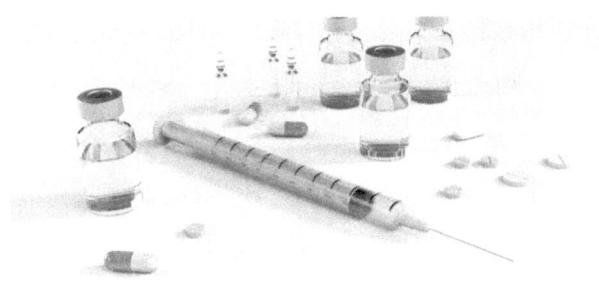

VITAMIN C - INTRAVENOUS

IV Vitamin C against viral infection

Vitamin C promotes the growth and spread of lymphocytes, a type of immune cell that increases circulating antibodies - proteins which can attack harmful viruses in the body. There is also some evidence from ongoing clinical trials in humans that high doses of intravenous vitamin C can reduce lung inflammation in severe respiratory illnesses that are caused by various pathogens and viruses. The use of vitamins boosted the activity of phagocytes which are immune cells that can destroy harmful viruses in the body.

Vitamin C is also one of the well-known antiviral agents, especially to influenza virus. It has shown its effect on antiviral immune responses through increased production of interferon at the early stage of infection - especially against influenza virus,

Worldwide clinical trials

Dr Richard Cheng MD, PhD, Chinese Edition Editor of the Orthomolecular Medicine News Service has written about ongoing clinical trials using Vitamin C for the treatment of viruses with encouraging results.

1. There were three clinical trials in China studying the effects of high-dose intravenous (IV) vitamin C for the treatment of viruses.

2. Dr. Cheng said that the Shanghai Medical Association has released a statement on the comprehensive treatment of viral infections where they endorsed the use of high-dose IV vitamin C.

3. Dr. Cheng said that a "Shanghai Plan" published on March 1, 2020 is the only official government guideline for using vitamin C for all kinds of viral infections.

4. He mentioned that some Chinese hospital groups are studying the effect of oral liposomal vitamin C for the treatments of viruses.

5. He thinks that this oral form of vitamin C can be administered rapidly to virus-infected patients.

6. Dr. Cheng's studies reveal that the preliminary results of the study were promising. His usage of 24 grams per day of vitamin C IV to patients lead to significant reductions in viral inflammation.

GENERAL REFERENCES:

Padayatty SJ, Katz A, Wang Y, Eck P, Kwon O, Lee JH, Chen S, Corpe C, Dutta A, Dutta SK, Levine M. Vitamin C as an antioxidant: evaluation of its role in disease prevention. J Am Coll Nutr. 2003;22:18–35.

Kojo S. Vitamin C: basic metabolism and its function as an index of oxidative stress. Curr Med Chem. 2004;11:1041–1064.

Boyera N, Galey I, Bernard BA. Effect of vitamin C and its derivatives on collagen synthesis and cross-linking by normal human fibroblasts. Int J Cosmet Sci. 1998;20:151–158.

Englard S, Seifter S. The biochemical functions of ascorbic acid. Annu Rev Nutr. 1986;6:365–406.

Noh K, Lim H, Moon SK, Kang JS, Lee WJ, Lee D, Hwang YI. Mega-dose Vitamin C modulates T cell functions in Balb/c mice only when administered during T cell activation. Immunol Lett. 2005;98:63–72.

Wintergerst ES, Maggini S, Hornig DH. Immune-enhancing role of vitamin C and zinc and effect on clinical conditions. Ann Nutr Metab. 2006;50:85–94.

Linster CL, Van Schaftingen E. Vitamin C. Biosynthesis, recycling and degradation in mammals. FEBS J. 2007;274:1–22.

Maeda N, Hagihara H, Nakata Y, Hiller S, Wilder J, Reddick R. Aortic wall damage in mice unable to synthesize ascorbic acid. Proc Natl Acad Sci U S A. 2000;97:841–846.

Kim H, Bae S, Yu Y, Kim Y, Kim HR, Hwang YI, Kang JS, Lee WJ. The analysis of vitamin C concentration in organs of gulo(-/-) mice upon vitamin C withdrawal. Immune Netw. 2012;12:18–26.

Bae S, Cho CH, Kim H, Kim Y, Kim HR, Hwang YI, Yoon JH, Kang JS, Lee WJ. In Vivo

Consequence of Vitamin C Insufficiency in Liver Injury: Vitamin C Ameliorates T-Cell-Mediated Acute Liver Injury in Gulo(-/-) Mice. Antioxid. Redox Signal. 2013

Pauling L. The significance of the evidence about ascorbic acid and the common cold. Proc Natl Acad Sci U S A. 1971;68:2678–2681.

Hemilä H, Chalker E. Vitamin C for preventing and treating the common cold. Cochrane Database Syst Rev. 2013;1:CD000980. doi: 10.1002/14651858.CD000980.pub4.

Hwang I, Scott JM, Kakarla T, Duriancik DM, Choi S, Cho C, Lee T, Park H, French AR, Beli E, Gardner E, Kim S. Activation mechanisms of natural killer cells during influenza virus infection. PLoS One. 2012;7:e51858. doi: 10.1371/journal.pone.0051858.

Zhou NN, Senne DA, Landgraf JS, Swenson SL, Erickson G, Rossow K, Liu L, Yoon KJ, Krauss S, Webster RG. Genetic reassortment of avian, swine, and human influenza A viruses in American pigs. J Virol. 1999;73:8851–8856.

Müller U, Steinhoff U, Reis LF, Hemmi S, Pavlovic J, Zinkernagel RM, Aguet M. Functional role of type I and type II interferons in anti-viral defense. Science. 1994;264:1918–1921.

Trinchieri G. Type I interferon: friend or foe? J Exp Med. 2010;207:2053–2063.

Horvath CM. The Jak-STAT pathway stimulated by interferon gamma. Sci STKE. 2004;2004:tr8.

Darnell JE, Jr, Kerr IM, Stark GR. Jak-STAT pathways and transcriptional activation in response to IFNs and other extracellular signaling proteins. Science. 1994;264:1415–1421.

Gongora C, Mechti N. Interferon signaling pathways. Bull Cancer. 1999;86:911–919.

Aymard-Henry M, Coleman MT, Dowdle WR, Laver WG, Schild GC, Webster RG. Influenzavirus neuraminidase and neuraminidase-inhibition test procedures. Bull World Health Organ. 1973;48:199–202.

Jack D. Warner

PROTOCOL 5

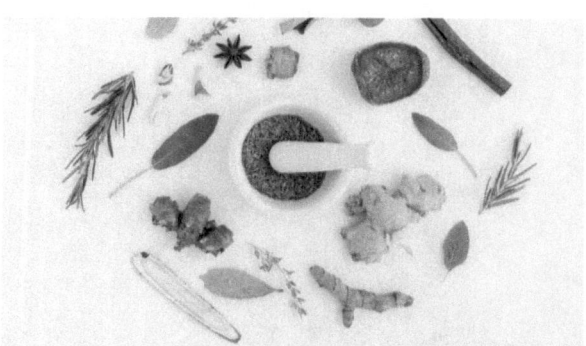

ANTIVIRAL HERBS LIST

Most common antiviral herbs which I consume as tea, capsules, and tincture.

1. CURCUMIN

Curcumin has a preventative and therapeutic role in viral infection and cytokine storms common to all viral infections.

2. SAGE

Sweet and holly varieties may fight certain viral infections. They have been shown to increase immunity, which may help fight viral infections.

3. OREGANO

Oregano of the mint family is known for its medicinal qualities. Its plant compounds, which include carvacrol, offer antiviral properties.

4. LEMON BALM

Lemon balm has been shown to have antiviral effects against avian influenza (bird flu), herpes viruses, HIV-1, and enterovirus 71.

5. GARLIC

Garlic may have antiviral activity against influenza A and B, HIV, viral pneumonia, and rhinovirus which may indicate that garlic enhances the immune system response by stimulating protective immune cells, which may safeguard against viral infections.

6. FENNEL

Fennel extract exhibited strong antiviral effects against herpes viruses and parainfluenza type-3, which causes respiratory infections in cattle

7. ELDERBERRY (SAMBUCUS)

Elderberry in a review of 4 studies in 180 people were found to substantially reduce upper respiratory symptoms caused by viral infections.

There Is data that suggests elderberry can reduce flu virus production and help people recover from the flu faster. A study published in March 2019 in the Journal of Functional Foods found that compounds from elderberries can inhibit the virus's entry and replication in human cells and help strengthen a person's immune response to the virus.

8. ROSEMARY

Oleanolic acid in Rosemary has displayed antiviral activity against herpes viruses, HIV, and hepatitis in animal and test-tube studies.

9. ECHINACEA

Echinacea is thought to have immune-boosting effects. It is also particularly useful for treating viral infections.

10. PEPPERMINT

Peppermint is known to contain active components, including menthol and rosmarinic acid, which have antiviral and anti-inflammatory activity.

11. LICORICE

Licorice root extract was effective against HIV, herpes viruses, and severe acute respiratory syndrome-related SARS-CoV, which causes a serious type of pneumonia.

12. ASTRAGALUS

Astragalus combats herpes viruses, hepatitis C, and avian influenza H9 virus. It plays an extraordinary role in lengthening our telomeres.

13. GINGER

Ginger extract has antiviral effects against avian influenza, and feline calicivirus, which is comparable to human norovirus. It also has been found to inhibit viral replication and prevent viruses from entering host cells.

14. GINSENG

Korean red ginseng extract has exhibited significant effects against herpes viruses, and hepatitis A.

15. DANDELION

Dandelion may combat hepatitis B, HIV, and influenza.

16. OLIVE LEAVES

The leaves of olive trees have been identified as powerful inhibitors of a wide range of viruses in laboratory tests., including influenza, herpes, polio and coxsackie viruses. These substances block the production of enzymes that allow viruses to replicate.

17. PAU D'ARCO

Pau d'arco is a tree said to have healing inner bark containing quinoids which inhibit virus replication by damaging the DNA and RNA inside the viral protein - the same viral protein that would normally insert itself in a healthy human cell and replicate.

18. CINNAMON

Its active compound which is called cinnamaldehyde has antiviral, immunomodulatory, antimicrobial, and anti-inflammatory effects. It also inhibits the growth of the influenza virus.

19. PELARGONIUM SIDOIDES

According to nih.com website this plant's extract alleviates symptoms of acute viral respiratory infections, including the common cold and bronchitis.

20. ANDROGRAPHIS PANICULATA

This herb contains andrographolide, a terpenoid compound found to have antiviral effects against respiratory-disease-causing viruses, including enterovirus D68 and influenza A.

GENERAL REFERENCES:

https://www.liebertpub.com/doi/abs/10.1089/act.2017.29150.eya

20 of the Best Antiviral and Antibacterial Herbs and Plants Ever! [Internet]. NaturalON – Natural Health News and Discoveries. 2015 [cited 2017Sep12]. Available from: http://naturalon.com/20-of-the-best-antiviral-and-antibacterial-herbs-and-plants-ever/view-all/

Goolsby J. 11 Anti-Viral Herbs for Fighting HPV [Internet]. Dr. Axe. 2017 [cited 2017Sep12]. Available from: https://draxe.com/how-to-treat-hpv/

https://timesofindia.indiatimes.com/life-style/health-fitness/home-remedies/6-anti-viral-herbs-that-will-help-you-stay-healthy/photostory/75386621.cms?picid=75386644

7 Anti-Viral Foods That Will Keep You Healthy Year-Round [Internet]. Natural Living Ideas. 2016 [cited 2017Sep12]. Available from: http://www.naturallivingideas.com/anti-viral-foods/

Human papillomavirus (HPV) and cervical cancer [Internet]. World Health Organization. World Health Organization; 2016 [cited 2017Sep12]. Available from: http://www.who.int/mediacentre/factsheets/fs380/en/

Jack D. Warner

PROTOCOL 6

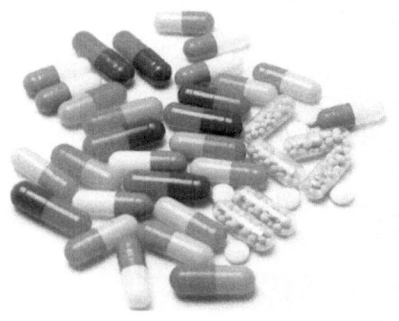

ANTIVIRAL SUPPLEMENTS

Here are some of my favorite and effective antiviral supplements.

VITAMIN D3

There is compelling evidence for an epidemiological association between poor vitamin D status and a variety of diseases. Clinical results in Medical Virology Volume 29, Issue 2 indicate a complex interplay between viral infections and vitamin D, including the induction of an antiviral state, functional immunoregulatory features, interaction with cellular and viral factors, induction of autophagy and apoptosis, and genetic and epigenetic alterations.

ZINC ACETATE

According to recent scientific studies zinc has been proven to be an essential micronutrient for the immune system to function. According to many clinical trials, supplementing with zinc may help protect against pneumonia. It has a role in antibody and white blood cell production and fights infections, while zinc deficiency increases inflammation and decreases the production of antibodies.

The best kind is zinc acetate. It is the only kind of zinc that consistently slashes the duration of inflammation in half. Why is zinc acetate effective and other kinds are not? Because they both release zinc in the form of a positively charged ion. The ionic form is what makes the difference in whether zinc can work or not. How does ionic zinc work? Well, ionic zinc helps the white blood cells fight. It boosts their production of interferon-gamma, which is one's body's primary defense. Ionic zinc also stops viral invaders from spreading in the body.

N-ACETYL-L-CYSTEINE (NAC)

N-acetyl-L-cysteine (NAC) is mentioned at the Clinicaltrials.gov website that researchers think that N-acetylcysteine can help fight the viruses by boosting a type of cell in the immune system that attacks infections. The anti-inflammatory and antioxidant effects in a number of pulmonary diseases have produced positive results in viral pneumonia and acute respiratory distress syndrome.

Recent clinical studies have revealed that NAC has increased the inhibitory effects on virus replication and production of pro-inflammatory molecules. The researchers believe that antioxidants like NAC represent a potential additional treatment option that could be considered in the case of an influenza A virus pandemic.

PROTEOLYTIC ENZYMES

Proteolytic enzymes have been proven to be lifesavers. Latest scientific studies have suggested that those enzymes have helped in the breakup of the dangerous clotting protein clusters that have accumulated in the endothelial blood vessel cells of virus-stricken patients.

Proteolytic enzymes are sold by many vitamin companies as prophylactic supplements to prevent the formation of blood clotting protein clusters in the blood vessels. The most known enzymes are Serrapeptase, Lumbrokinase and Nattokinase. I have been taking Serrapeptase supplements for quite some time now.

GENERAL REFERENCES:

https://onlinelibrary.wiley.com/toc/10991654/2019/29/2

https://clinicaltrials.gov/ct2/show/NCT04374461

https://clinicaltrials.gov/ct2/show/NCT04335084

https://www.sciencedirect.com/science/article/abs/pii/S000629520900728X?via%3Dihub

https://www.healthline.com/nutrition/vitamin-d-coronavirus

The Scientist November 3, 2020

U.S. News & World Report July 23, 2020

International Journal of Surgery, 2013 Apr;11(3):209-217

Scientific Reports 2015; 5: 11601

Jack D. Warner

PROTOCOL 7

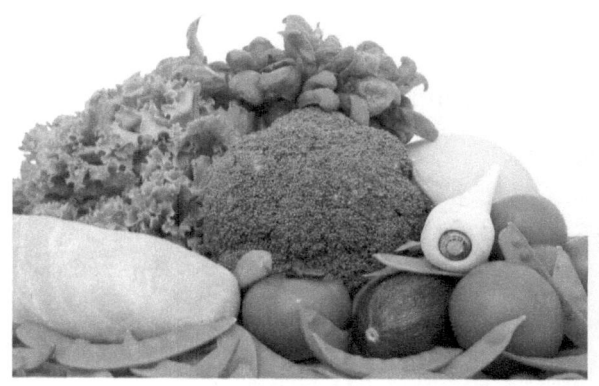

ANTIVIRAL FOOD

Yes, there really is something called antiviral food that helps in maintaining an optimum immune system in the fight against viral inflammations. The followings are foods for strengthening the immune system.

SHIITAKE MUSHROOMS

1. They contain Beta-glucans which is one of the most supporting immune systems. The beta-glucans are sugars that have antiviral capabilities. In fact, hospitals administer beta-glucans via IVs to prevent infection post-surgery.

2. They have been shown to inhibit viral replication.

3. They have significant antibacterial and antifungal properties,

4. They are a great source of copper. Copper helps the body increase the number of T cells which work to fight off infections.

5. They also help the body create new antibodies which are useful in combating infections.

6. One study on the antiviral benefits of shiitake mushrooms found that these foods had a positive impact on the immune system. Researchers stated that compounds in shiitake mushrooms increased secretory immunoglobulin A in the body

APPLE CIDER VINEGAR

The mother of apples form of organic apple cider vinegar has antiviral properties and is also rich in probiotics that is produced from the fermentation process. Acetic acid in vinegar is effective in combating antifungal, antibacterial and antiviral diseases.

YOGURT

One of the best antiviral foods is probiotics. Probiotics in yogurt help the gut against viral infection. Filling the gut biome with good bacteria has shown to help fight off the growth of enterovirus.

Yogurt which is naturally rich in probiotics can protect against respiratory tract infections. Also, it has been shown to lessen the severity of respiratory infections that is caused by the influenza virus.

BELL PEPPERS

Bell peppers are known to boost the immune system by the presence of vitamin C which helps the body create new white blood cells that work naturally to ward off infections.

OYSTERS

Oysters are one of the foods that have the highest amount of zinc mineral that promotes immune T cells maturation and performance,

SWEET POTATOES

Sweet potatoes are rich in carbohydrates and fiber that are good for gut health. They are rich in vitamin A which plays an important role in the structure and function of B and T cells.

TUNA

Tuna is an excellent source of vitamin B6.

1. This vitamin is an enhancer to the immune system,
2. It plays a crucial role in building antibodies.
3. It regulates inflammation within the body.

BLACK TEA

Black tea leaves contain pathogen-fighting polyphenols, catechins, and alkaloids such as caffeine, theobromine, and theophylline that can protect against a variety of viral infections such as the influenza virus.

Black tea extract is also rich in flavanol compounds called theaflavins which is effective in inhibiting herpes simplex virus type-1 infection.

GREEN TEA

EGCG, (Epigallocatechin 3-Galate) the most abundant catechin in green tea, was shown to minimize the infectivity of the influenza A and B virus in kidney cells. Furthermore, EGCG inhibited the activity of viral RNA (ribonucleic acid), which suppressed virus propagation.

GENERAL REFERENCES

https://pubmed.ncbi.nlm.nih.gov/25866155/

https://www.ncbi.nlm.nih.gov/pmc/articles/PMC6100025/

https://www.ncbi.nlm.nih.gov/pmc/articles/PMC3217690/

https://link.springer.com/article/10.1007/s10068-010-0042-x

https://blog.thryveinside.com/probiotic-foods-bacteria-in-yogurt/

https://www.ncbi.nlm.nih.gov/pmc/articles/PMC6100025/

https://www.ncbi.nlm.nih.gov/pmc/articles/PMC3217690/

https://pubmed.ncbi.nlm.nih.gov/25866155/

Kill Viruses Now

PROTOCOL 8

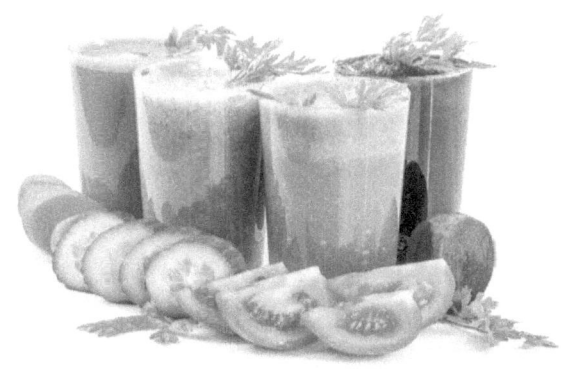

IMMUNE BOOSTING JUICES

My Favorite Antiviral Juices that I consume daily. I try to combine different ingredients according to my taste.

GRAPEFRUIT

The juice of grapefruit has tremendous antiviral properties. It contains a substance called maringin that boosts up the body's metabolic function. A strong metabolism often ensures better immunity and resistance to common viral infection.

LEMON

Lemon has tremendous antiviral properties because of the presence of vitamin C.

ONION

Onion is a very strong antiseptic, antiviral, and antibiotic food. Onion is especially rich in quercetin that has a broad range of antiviral activity. It is known among scientists for its ability to intervene at multiple steps of pathogen virulence, including inhibiting virus entry, replication, and protein assembly.

DILL

Dill is a leafy green with various health benefits. The herb is well known for its antiviral properties. Dill is known to cure stomach flu and also viral infections like influenza.

STAR ANISE

It is one of the best antiviral foods. It has been used since ancient times as an herbal medicine for improving the immune function. This licorice-flavored spice is rich in shikimic acid. Shikimic acid has potent antiviral properties. It is also an active ingredient in Theraflu!

OLIVE LEAVES

Olive leaves are one of the most abundant sources of oleuropein. Studies involving this molecule found that it shows significant effects against respiratory virus and parainfluenza type 3 virus.

SPIRULINA

One study showed the effects of spirulina inhibiting virus replication. Many of the antiviral benefits of spirulina are attributed to its high levels of cyanovirin-N. This protein has been shown to slow down the progression of HIV and AIDS. It is also shown promise in blocking the progression of the herpes simplex virus type-1.

GENERAL REFERENCES

https://www.ncbi.nlm.nih.gov/pmc/articles/PMC3002804/

https://pubmed.ncbi.nlm.nih.gov/15000694/

https://www.euroformhealthcare.biz/human-nutrition/spirulina-antiviral-studies-in-vivo.html

https://pubmed.ncbi.nlm.nih.gov/15869811/

https://heatherdane.com/star-anise-for-utis-flu-digestion-and-viral-infections/

https://howtocure.com/health-benefits-of-dill/

https://www.google.com/search?client=firefox-b-1-d&q=pathogen+virulence

https://www.wellnessresources.com/studies/grape-seed-extracts-anti-viral-activity

Jack D. Warner

PROTOCOL 9

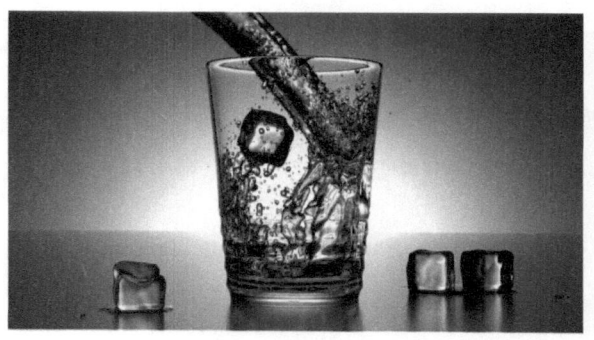

NITRIC OXIDE(NO)

What is nitric oxide?

Nitric Oxide, which is known also as NO, is an important signaling molecule in the body that exists in the form of a gas; it is made up of just one molecule of nitrogen and just one molecule of oxygen. NO is produced in several places in the body, but mostly in the endothelium lining of the blood vessels.

How does nitric oxide help the body?

Nitric Oxide performs many important functions in the body.

1. It helps blood vessels dilate.

2. It promotes proper circulation and blood flow to the arteries of the heart.

3. It improves exercise performance.

4. It lowers blood pressure.

5. It improves brain function.

6. It improves symptoms of clogged arteries and angina.

7. It boosts energy and sexual performance.

8. It can reduce the number of virus-infected cells by hundreds of times.

9. It can give crucial support to the lungs by helping breathing deeply.

10. It also can reduce pulmonary artery pressure thus resulting in maintaining oxygen supply to their lungs.

How can we supply the body with nitric oxide?

Nitric oxide can be easily induced by the body within ten minutes by consuming certain combinations of amino acids.

CITRULLINE MALATE

Citrulline malate is commonly found in watermelons, while malate is derived from the Latin word for apple. This amino acid has a long history of use in sports nutrition because of its ability to influence nitric oxide production in the body.

L-GLYCINE

L-Glycine is an amino acid that helps lower heart disease risk factors by increasing the body's ability to use nitric oxide.

AAKG

Arginine-alpha-ketoglutarate (AAKG) supplements are known to increase nitric oxide production resulting in vasodilation.

L-TAURINE

L-Taurine is known to causes vascular relaxation through the modulation of endothelium-derived nitric oxide. It has antiarrhythmic properties resulting from its role as a nitric oxide (NO) precursor.

There are other amino acids that also have the property of inducing NO in the body to a lesser extent. I usually combine all the above mentioned amino acids in this section and take them as needed either in the mornings and/or evenings for therapeutic dosage of Nitric Oxide.

GENERAL REFERENCES

https://www.ncbi.nlm.nih.gov/pmc/articles/PMC6164974/

Bradford M.M. A rapid and sensitive method for the quantitation of microgram quantities of protein utilizing the principle of protein-dye binding. Anal. Biochem. 1976;72:248–254. doi: 10.1016/0003-2697(76)90527-3.

Panza J.A., Quyyumi A.A., Brushm J.E., Jr., Epstein S.E. Abnormal endothelium-dependent vascular relaxation in patients with essential hypertension. N. Engl. J. Med. 1990;323:22–27. doi: 10.1056/NEJM199007053230105.

https://www.ncbi.nlm.nih.gov/pmc/articles/PMC6164974/

https://pubmed.ncbi.nlm.nih.gov/30847640/

https://www.bodybuilding.com/content/6-evidence-based-benefits-of-citrulline-malate.html

https://www.healthline.com/nutrition/glycine

https://pubmed.ncbi.nlm.nih.gov/21813912/

https://www.ncbi.nlm.nih.gov/pmc/articles/PMC3268940/

https://www.sciencedirect.com/science/article/abs/pii/S1089860319302113

https://pubmed.ncbi.nlm.nih.gov/16797868/

Kill Viruses Now

CONCLUSION

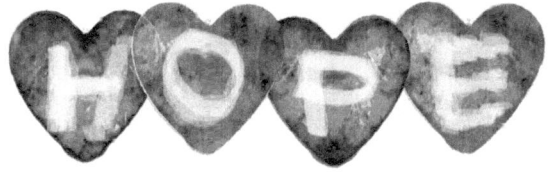

I hope you have enjoyed this introduction of my therapeutic protocols. I have enjoyed sharing my knowledge with you. As I have mentioned in the preface, this book and the subsequent books in Health and Wellness Series have been inspired by the prodding of my friends, and personal physicians.

I am looking forward to publishing Volume 2 under the title name of PERFECT DE-AGING which deals with reversing old age. Volume 3 titled INCREDIBLE SHAKES OF THE GODS introduces the most delicious and comprehensive therapeutic shakes of all times.

Please notice that the general references in this book are provided to give readers a chance to explore for themselves more information on the latest fight against ancient and novel viral diseases.

Detailed information about the updates of my protocols will be accessible through my Amazon Author's Page here: https://author.amazon.com/home

I sincerely wish you and your family the healthiest and the happiest life ever! I do hope that you found this book or parts of it beneficial.

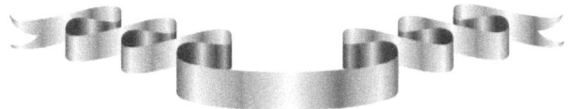

Jack D. Warner

Coming Soon - Volume 2

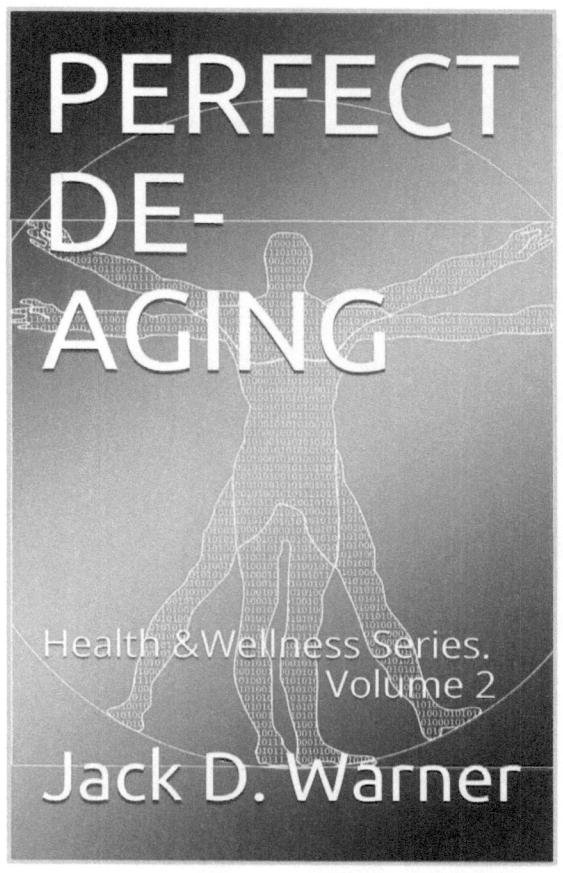

PERFECT DE-AGING

This book is the culmination of all my latest exciting scientific discoveries into life extension and rejuvenation. It covers a lot of natural treatments that delve into the realm of the successful reversal of what is normally considered to be the inevitable aging process and its dire consequences. Aging is a disease as many scientists are now claiming. Aging could be delayed, stopped, or even reversed.

In this book you will discover all the incredible natural treatments that I have been using with great success. I am the living proof that there is a cure for the disease of old age.

Jack D. Warner

Coming Soon - Volume 3

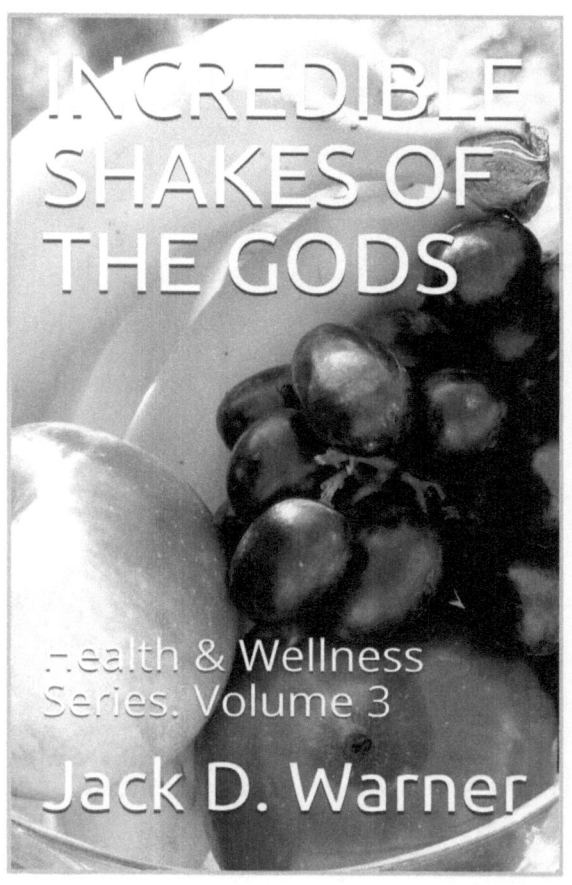

Kill Viruses Now

INCREDIBLE SHAKES OF THE GODS

This book contains exciting recipes for optimum health and rejuvenation. The recipes are geared towards providing innovative healing shakes that would supply vigor and vitality to every parts of the body. This would include support for the brain, eyes, skin, all internal organs, moods, and mental health.

This book is divided into many categories that deal with problems that the individual wants to correct through specially designed shakes that would target the healing and correction of the specific physical, psychological and spiritual impediments in question.

Jack D. Warner

About the Author

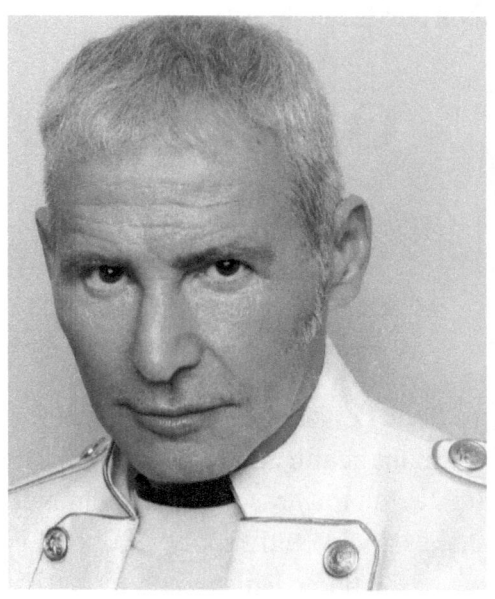

Jack D Warner has worked as a professor at various Colleges and Universities in Southern California, USA. He has been loved and respected by everyone for his optimistic lifestyle that made him sound, act and look like a youthful person half of his biological age. Jack's secrets are finally out since his recent decision to share his greatest health accomplishments with the whole world. It has been a known fact of the great interest of his physicians and friends to have Jack write a book about what he does in order to keep himself super-healthy and rejuvenated all the time.

Jack has been an avid follower of his own made-up protocols of healthy healing food and advanced supplementations for decades. Alas, during the past few years, he never had the will to make known the details of his protocols until he started to write his Health and Wellness Series. Finally, Jack's complete honesty in the revelation of the alleged secrets of his incredible sustenance and healthy longevity is a refreshing addition towards a disease-free world. He seems to have stumbled upon something unique that teeter on the supernatural. He seems to always zoom in on the latest scientific discoveries in the field of rejuvenation and health with the purpose of applying them on himself. Jack's life seems to miraculously evolve toward defeating old age and its accompanying miseries. Perhaps Jack's physicians' curiosity about his sustainable perfect health and rejuvenation proves beyond any doubts the practicability and viability of his healing protocols.

Please review this book if you find it beneficial. Thank you!

www.ingramcontent.com/pod-product-compliance
Lightning Source LLC
Chambersburg PA
CBHW020445220526
45464CB00002B/865